M000032488

the little book of
YOGA

Published by OH!
20 Mortimer Street
London W1T 3JW

Disclaimer:
This book and the information contained herein are for general educational and entertainment use only. The contents are not claimed to be exhaustive, and the book is sold on the understanding that neither the publishers nor the author are thereby engaged in rendering any kind of professional services. Users are encouraged to confirm the information contained herein with other sources and review the information carefully with their appropriate, qualified service providers. Neither the publishers nor the author shall have any responsibility to any person or entity regarding any loss or damage whatsoever, direct or indirect, consequential, special or exemplary, caused or alleged to be caused, by the use or misuse of information contained in this book.

ISBN 978-1-91161-069-4

Editorial consultant: Sasha Fenton
Editorial: Fiona Channon, Victoria Godden
Project manager: Russell Porter
Design: Ben Ruocco
Production: Rachel Burgess

A CIP catalogue record for this book is available from the British Library

Printed in China

10 9 8 7 6 5 4 3

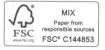

MIX
Paper from
responsible sources
FSC® C144853
www.fsc.org

Illustrations: Tond Van Graphcraft/Shutterstock, piixypeach/Freepik

the little book of
YOGA

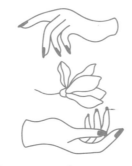

fiona channon

CONTENTS

INTRODUCTION

The word yoga is derived from Sanskrit and means "union". This refers to the union of mind and body achieved through a series of postures or exercises called asanas that stretch, tone and strengthen the body. Most poses have names that end in the word "asana". For example: "Gomukhasana", which means "Cow Pose". You won't be expected to remember the names, and you shouldn't allow the Sanskrit to put you off. Incidentally, a person who does yoga is called a yogi.

Yoga was originally invented to balance and harmonize the mind, body and emotions, and was used as a preparation for meditation. For a lot of people, meditation is not only misunderstood, but it doesn't appeal, and this may have stopped them from trying yoga as a result.

The good news, however, is that the benefits of the poses, are so numerous that a lot of people have started to do yoga as part of their keep-fit regime or simply to feel good. It's only after a period of time doing yoga that you realize your attitude and demeanour may have changed for the better, and it will have done so in a natural manner.

There are two sides to yoga: one is the physical and the other is spiritual and subtle, but you can still do yoga for the physical benefits even if you're not interested in learning about the spiritual aspects.

If you are not physically completely fit, it would be advisable to start practising yoga with a professional teacher, so that you don't accidentally overreach your body's exercise limits. When you know your safe levels of exertion, you can then continue on your own at home.

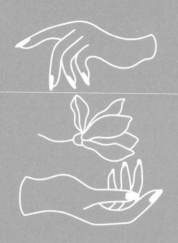

CHAPTER

1

DEBUNKING the MYTHS around YOGA

I'M NOT FLEXIBLE ENOUGH TO DO YOGA

That's the whole point! If you're not flexible, you need yoga, which will start to stretch the body so that you become more supple.

IT FEELS
LIKE A CULT

Unfortunately there's a stigma attached to yoga from the old days. It seemed mystical and almost religious – but it really isn't.

If you approach it as simply part of your exercise regime, you won't feel so intimidated by it.

I'M TOO UNFIT

You can only start with what you have. It doesn't matter how fit you are, you just have to start at the beginning. Give yourself a chance.

I'M TOO OLD

Tao Porchon-Lynch, the Guinness-certified world's oldest yoga teacher, died at age 101! She had a wonderful philosophy about life and didn't let age stop her. She did yoga her whole life, demonstrating that age is no more than a state of mind.

I'M TOO FAT

It doesn't matter what size you are,
because you can always do something.
Besides, doing yoga can actually help you
to lose weight.

IT'S FOR HIPPIES

Most of the people who come to my classes are perfectly normal people of all ages, shapes and sizes. I'll admit that some hippies are attracted to yoga, but don't let that put you off. Besides, hippies are usually lovely people.

Everyone else
KNOWS WHAT
they're doing
AND I DON'T

It may seem that way, but I can assure you they don't. There may be some people in your class with more experience, but they are not trying to make you feel bad, because they are there for themselves. If they are experienced, they'll know that you will get there when you're ready.

I'M TOO SELF-CONSCIOUS and EMBARRASSED

It can be nerve-wracking going to a new class to do something you've never done before. If you go with an open mind and heart and forget about how you look, you will get far more out of it than you can imagine. Everyone is on their own journey.

I'VE GOT A DODGY KNEE

Obviously, you always need to take your doctor's advice if you have a medical issue, but you can work around injuries. If you have a bad knee, then work with the good one, or some poses (asanas) can be adjusted or adapted to suit you better. As long as you tell your teacher, they can help you find a more suitable adaptation.

It's for young,
FIT PEOPLE
with tattoos and
TOPKNOTS

There are a few of those, I'll admit, but there are also a lot of older people joining classes yjese days. The range of ages in my classes is from seventeen to seventy-four. This is where one must avoid being judgemental, because we all have something to learn.

I'M NOT
INTERESTED
in SPIRITUALITY

You don't have to be into spirituality to enjoy yoga. You might hear the odd Sanskrit word, but it's not compulsory to know about the more esoteric side of yoga unless you want to – you can just approach it as exercise if that's what you prefer.

IT'S AGAINST MY RELIGION

Yoga is a philosophy with a physical practice. Yoga philosophy stems from a system that predates Hinduism but which influenced it, thus the similarities. But whereas Hinduism is a religion, yoga is not; it is practised by people of many religions and others who are secular.

to SUMMARIZE

Hopefully, this first chapter will have countered some of your resistance to trying a yoga class. Remember: everything is optional.

"When you own your breath, nobody can steal your peace."

ANONYMOUS

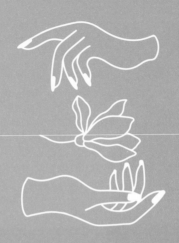

CHAPTER

2

MAKING a START

WHAT HAPPENS in a YOGA CLASS

You will be greeted by the yoga teacher and made to feel welcome.

Remove your footwear (yoga is done barefoot), and find a spot to place your mat. If you don't have a mat, ask the teacher if there is one you can borrow.

Leave a good amount of space between you and the next person, as you will be stretching out your arms and legs and you don't want to touch the person next to you if you can help it.

The teacher will introduce the session and tell you how to start.

This usually involves gathering yourself first by focusing the mind, so take a few deep breaths (either lying down or sitting) to bring the energy into the body and find stillness.

The teacher will then take you through a series of postures (asanas) with breaks between each one to allow you to integrate what you've just done.

You will be told to use the breath with the posture, and will spend time working on each part of the body.

Remember to listen to your body and come out of a pose if it's too difficult.

Just before the end of the session, there are usually some breathing exercises which help to relax the mind even more in preparation for the last part of the class.

Many students consider this the best bit, because it is the relaxation section.

At the end of the session, after the breathing, you will feel ready to go into the relaxation segment of the class, which is wonderful after doing the poses, and the teacher will talk you through a relaxation process.

This is called Savasana, which means "Corpse Pose", where you lie on your back with your feet flopped open and hands palm up on the floor by your hips.

PROPS
and EQUIPMENT

Some sports and exercise systems can cost a fortune, but yoga isn't one of them. Yoga is as much about the mind and spirit as it is the body, so don't be seduced by expensive gear that you don't need and may not be able to afford. However, if you want more kit as you go along, you might be able to find used items on the internet. You don't have to buy any equipment to start with, and the props that I list here are optional.

YOGA MAT

Essentially all you need is a mat that is called a sticky mat. It creates traction for your hands and feet so you don't slip if you get a little sweaty. It also provides cushioning on a hard floor. Most yoga teachers have spare mats but it's good to have your own if you know you're going to continue.

If you're not sure about whether you are going to keep going with your yoga class, use the teacher's mats for a few weeks and see how you feel.

By the way, it is considered impolite to step on someone else's mat unless they've invited you on. It's a matter of hygiene for those with bare feet.

BLANKETS

The final part of the yoga session is where you lie down to relax the body, and this is called Savasana. Some say it's the best bit, and can sometimes involve snoring! The body temperature drops when we stop moving, so a blanket keeps you warm and enables you to stay relaxed during this part of the session.

BLOCKS

These are used to make you comfortable and improve your alignment. Blocks are particularly useful for standing poses in which your hands are supposed to be on the floor. Placing a block under your hand has the effect of "raising the floor" to meet your hand rather than forcing the hand to come to the floor, which could cause injury or reduce the benefits of the pose.

"The yoga mat is a good place to turn to, when talk therapy and anti-depressants aren't enough."

AMY WEINTRAUB

CLOTHING

Although there are a lot of trendy and expensive yoga clothes out there, all you need to wear is something comfortable and loose that won't dig in when lying down or restrict your ability to move.

Apart from that it really doesn't matter what you wear. Anything goes.

YOGA SOCKS

To be clear, yoga socks are not a requirement, and it is actually preferable to do yoga barefoot. That said, if you get cramp or are uncomfortable barefoot, invest in a pair of yoga socks with grips on the bottom so you can keep your feet covered while maintaining good traction. Standard socks absolutely won't do and they can be dangerous, because they will make you slip.

STRAPS

Yoga straps, also called belts, are particularly useful for poses where you need to hold onto your feet but cannot reach them. The strap basically acts as an arm extender.

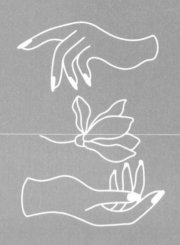

CHAPTER
3

DIFFERENT TYPES of YOGA

There are many types
of yoga, and trying to
work out which is which
can be overwhelming.
Each individual should
find a type of yoga most
suited to their needs, but
a good place to start is
Hatha yoga.

HATHA YOGA

If you are brand new to yoga, Hatha yoga is a great entry point to the practice. Hatha yoga classes are best for beginners, since they are usually paced more slowly than other yoga styles. This is the classic yoga, which involves the use of asanas (poses), pranayama (breath control), mudra (gestures) and bandha locks (which we will get to later in the book).

IYENGAR YOGA

Founded by B. K. S. Iyengar, Iyengar yoga focuses on alignment and detailed and precise movements. In an Iyengar class, students perform a variety of postures while controlling their breathing. Generally, poses are held for a long time, while adjusting the minutiae of the pose. Iyengar relies heavily on props to help students perfect their form and go deeper into poses in a safe manner. This style is really great for people with injuries who need to work slowly and methodically.

KUNDALINI
YOGA

This yoga practice is equal part spiritual and physical. It's all about releasing the spiritual energy in your body called Kundalini, which is said to be coiled in the lower spine. These classes really work your core, with fast-moving, invigorating postures and breathing exercises. These classes are pretty intense and can involve chanting, mantra and meditation.

ASHTANGA
YOGA

Ashtanga yoga involves a very physically demanding sequence of postures, so this style of yoga is definitely not for the beginner. It takes an experienced yogi to really love it. Ashtanga starts with ten Sun Salutations, which is a sequence of movements (shown on pages 64–65), and then moves into a series of standing and floor postures.

VINYASA YOGA

In Vinyasa classes, the movement is coordinated with your breath and movement to flow from one pose to another seamlessly. Commonly referred to as flow yoga, it is sometimes confused with power yoga. Vinyasa classes offer a variety of postures and no two classes are ever alike.

BIKRAM YOGA

Otherwise known as hot yoga, Bikram yoga features a sequence of set poses in a sauna-like room, which is typically set to 105 degrees and 40% humidity. The sequence includes a series of 26 basic postures, with each one performed twice. Many of these poses are focused on proper alignment. It's not so much that the yoga is hard, but you might find the heat a challenge. The idea is that the muscles are warmed up and you are less likely to injure yourself.

YIN
YOGA

Yin yoga targets the connective tissues
and joints of the body in a deep way. It's
a slow-paced style of yoga with seated
postures that are held for longer periods
of time. Yin is a great class for beginners,
as the classes are relaxed and you're
supposed to let gravity do most of the
work and feel amazing afterwards.
It also helps you to understand your own
body's resistance while in the poses.

NAAD
YOGA

The science of Naad yoga is the exploration of how sound vibrations affect the body, mind and spirit through the movement of the tongue and mouth, as well as chemical changes in the brain. Although it does involve an element of physical practice, Naad yoga is focused on finding wholeness through the use of devotional chanting and music.

RESTORATIVE YOGA

This yoga is wonderfully relaxing and excellent if you are suffering from burnout, helping you to cleanse and free your mind. Many props are used and these are placed to support the body so that you can just sink deeper into relaxation. Blankets, bolsters and eye pillows are commonly found in Restorative yoga sessions. You spend more time in each posture during the class, so there will be fewer of them.

GOAT, BEER
or ALPACA
YOGA

These are just fads, and although amusing, shouldn't be considered proper yoga classes. However, if you are in need of cheering up or want to try something new then by all means give them a go.

Did you know that there is also seated yoga for the disabled and elderly? Seated, or "chair", yoga is great for those who have medical conditions that prevent them from doing many of the classic Hatha yoga postures. If you are faced with issues of ageing combined with various aches and pains and challenges when standing or walking, this is the type of yoga for you. You may notice enough improvement to progress to some of the standing postures with the chair beside you after a time. Whatever your situation, moving the body is important.

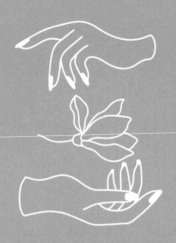

CHAPTER
4

ASANAS,
MUDRAS
and BANDHAS

ASANAS: POSES

Through holding the body in different asanas, or poses, your awareness of your own body is raised, which leads you to an understanding of yourself and the more subtle areas of existence, such as energy and stillness.

There are groups of asanas that are directed towards a certain part of the body and have many benefits. They strengthen, tone and mobilize the body.

On a more subtle level, they remove any blockages which prevent the free flow of energy in the body and mind. Yoga poses promote total health, regulating and balancing the flow of energy through the body.

"Yoga is 99% practice and 1% theory."

SRI KRISHNA PATTABHI JOIS

PRACTISING ASANAS

By practising these asanas, you will
be able to manage various disorders of
the body and maintain good health.
As well as opening up the major joints,
they will relax the muscles. Remember,
asanas should not be treated casually
just because they seem simple, gentle
or comfortable.

'Remember, it doesn't matter how deep into a posture you go, what does matter is who you are when you get there.'

MAX STROM

COUNTERPOSE

When practising the poses, it is important to do a counterpose. For example, a backward bend is followed by a forward bend, and vice versa, and whatever is practised on one side of the body is repeated on the other side. This is necessary to bring the body back to a balanced state.

"*Yoga is a dance between control and surrender, between pushing and letting go, and when to push and when to let go becomes part of the creative process, part of the open-ended exploration of your being.*"

JOEL KRAMER

asanas for
DEPRESSION

By moving the body and focusing on the breath during yoga, you are shifting sluggish energy around the body. Dynamic asanas, such as standing and twisting and back-bending ones that open the heart and chest, are good for depression, as well as a classic pose called "Sun Salutation" (see overleaf).

Sun Salutation

1.

2.

5.

6.

8.

9.

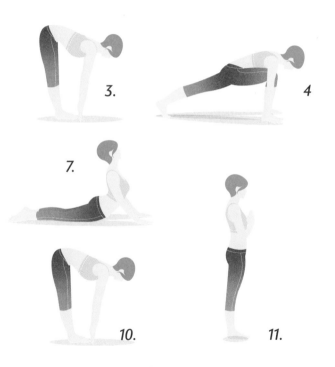

3.

4

7.

10.

11.

One good pose for depression is Setubandha Sarvangasana, otherwise known as Bridge Pose. To do this, lie on your back and bend the knees with your feet on the floor, but close to your bottom. Your palms should be face down on the floor beside your hips.

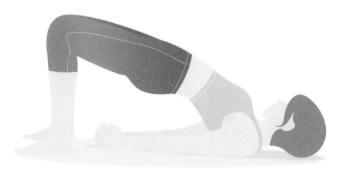

Bridge Pose

As you exhale, push your feet and arms actively into the floor. Push your tailbone upward toward the ceiling, and lift your buttocks off the floor. Keep your thighs and feet parallel.

Shuffle at the shoulders, bringing your shoulder blades towards each other, and interlace your fingers underneath your body. Push your chest up and keep your hands on the floor.

Stay in the pose anywhere from thirty seconds to one minute. Release with an exhalation, rolling your spine slowly down onto the floor.

asanas for
TRAUMA

Unfortunately most of us will experience trauma at some point in our lives. It can be a life-changing moment that either destroys or hardens us, leaving us numb and disassociated.

The emotions from that event get trapped in the body, but yoga can help you to release them through gentle practice. Recognize that the body has suffered a shock – and that it is continuing to suffer – so you must be kind to it and gentle, as you would be to a dear friend who is suffering. To overcome trauma, you need to do hip-opening and heart-opening poses.

A simple pose for trauma is Pond Pose,
or Tadagasana.

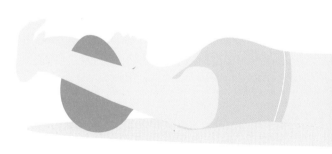

Pond Pose

Tightness in the diaphragm can be the result of panic. One asana for releasing trauma is to lie on your back with arms above your head and the backs of the hands resting on the mat. Stretching this way in the Pond Pose lengthens the abdominal cavity, opening the chest so that the diaphragm can move easily. When the breath is free, the nervous system is calm and we feel less desperation.

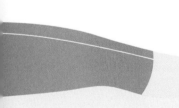

asanas for
DIGESTION

If you feel sluggish after overindulging, then doing a few yoga moves can help shift things along.

If you suffer from trapped wind or any other digestive issues, yoga can help, because there are certain asanas that can get the stomach working properly and assist with the movement of food through the intestines and bowel.

Squats, twists and lunges are great yoga moves to stimulate your digestive tract. Squatting gets everything moving downward, while twists massage the internal organs. Lunges help stretch the muscle that connects your body to your legs, and also the abdominal region, which aids in processing and eliminating food.

One simple asana for improved digestion is Ardha Pawamuktasana, also known as the Half Gas Release Pose.

Lie on your back and bring your right knee up to your chest, and hug it in.

Keep your left leg engaged by straightening it along the floor and pushing the heel away.

Hold the position for a few breaths and
then repeat with the left leg.

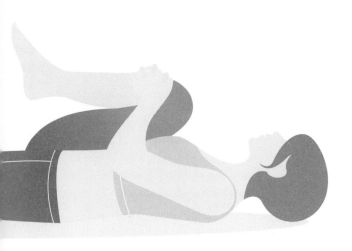

Half Gas Release Pose

asanas for
BACKACHE

Back pain costs the
UK economy £20 billion
every year!

Suffering with a bad back is no joke,
and it can be totally debilitating.

With regular practice, yoga can help
you to release stiffness and even
prevent surgery. It's always best to
check with your doctor first though,
depending on the issue.

Otherwise, use yoga to help you
maintain good spinal health and
mobility.

One good asana for backache is
Marjariasana, also known as the Cat-Cow
Pose.

Come down onto all fours on the mat.
Make sure the arms are under the
shoulders and knees are hip-width apart.
Inhale while raising your head, depressing
your spine and lifting your tail so that
your back becomes concave. Exhale while
lowering your head and curling your pelvis
under so that your back is arched.

Your head will now be between your arms
facing the thighs. Hold your breath for
three seconds for each inhale and exhale.
Do this a few times.

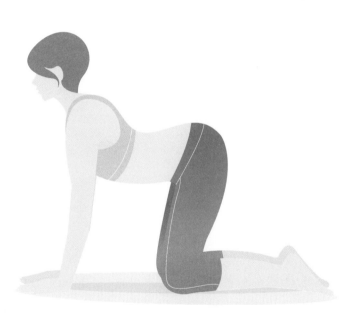

Cat-Cow Pose

asanas for
TIGHT HIPS

It's not very hard to find
someone with whom to
commiserate about hip pain,
because tight hips are right
up there with lower-back pain
and knee pain.

There are many potential causes, and sitting for several hours a day is commonly cited as the main source of hip tightness.

That's because when you sit all day, your hip muscles are forced into a shortened position for a long time.

Eventually, this can make them super tight, affecting your range of motion, which can impact everything from how deeply you can squat or lunge to the length of your running stride.

Tight hip flexors can also make it harder for your gluteus muscles to activate, which can lead other muscles to compensate and take on more work than they can handle, typically those in the lower back, thus increasing your risk of injury.

One easy asana for tight hips is Ananda Balasana, commonly known as Happy Baby Pose.

Lie on your back and bring your knees up to your chest. Bring your arms up on the inside of your knees and grab the outside of your feet.

Widen your legs to deepen the stretch.
Show the soles of your feet to the ceiling,
pulling your knees to your chest.

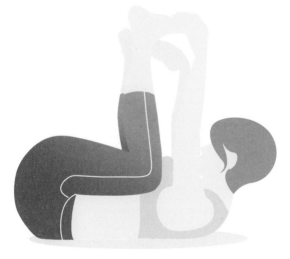

Happy Baby Pose

"Change only happens in the present moment. The past is already done. The future is just energy and intention."

KINO MacGREGOR

*"The yoga pose
you avoid the
most you need
the most."*

ANONYMOUS

asanas for tight
SHOULDERS

We store a lot of tension in our neck and shoulders and it's very hard to release once it has set in, which can lead to headaches or migraines.

Some simple neck and shoulder exercises can really help to release and prevent the development of a frozen shoulder.

Just sitting and breathing can also help you to relax and drop the shoulders, thus easing tension.

One yoga pose that's good for tight shoulders is Prasarita Padottanasana, commonly called Wide-Legged Forward Bend.

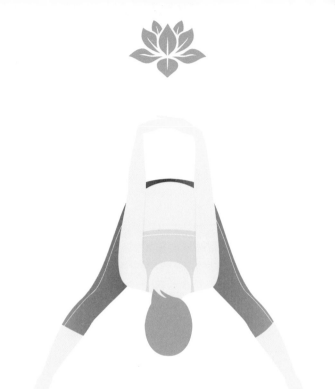

Wide-Legged Forward Bend

Stand with your feet wide apart, toes pointing forwards. Bring your hands behind your back and interlace your fingers. Bring your shoulder blades towards each other, inhale and fold forwards lifting your arms up behind you as far as they will go. Feel the stretch across the chest and in the shoulders. Focus on the breath. Slightly bend the knees as you come back up.

"I bend so I don't break."

ANONYMOUS

MUDRAS:
HAND
GESTURES

You may have seen pictures of people sitting cross-legged, with their hands on their knees and their fingers held in a certain shape and wondered why this is.

The pose that the hands are in is called a mudra. A mudra is a combination of subtle physical movements which alter mood, attitude and perception and which deepen awareness and concentration.

It may involve the whole body in a combination of pose, breath or visualization, or it may just be a simple hand position.

Mudras are usually introduced after the student has gained some proficiency.

FINGER GYM

It is possible to do yoga while sitting at your desk, or anywhere for that matter, using just your hands. You can gently try to bend the fingers back one at a time to open the joints and stretch them out. If you have arthritis, take care with such exercises. Moving your hands and fingers helps keep your ligaments and tendons flexible. Regular hand exercise strengthens muscles and relieves stiffness and pain.

BANDHAS

The word bandha is Sanskrit and means "to lock" or "to close-off". This describes the physical action (usually a muscular contraction), but the aim is to affect the energy in certain parts of the body. If you've ever squeezed your buttocks to stop yourself going to the loo, that is effectively a bandha.

The bandhas you will likely come across in a yoga class are the mula bandha, which affects the lowest part of the body, and the uddiyana bandha, which is pulling in the stomach to the spine. Your teacher will tell you when and how to do each bandha.

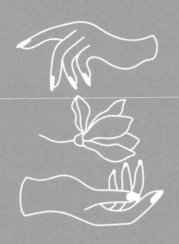

CHAPTER
5

the
BENEFITS
of YOGA

According to medical
scientists, yoga is
successful because it
creates balance in the
nervous and endocrine
systems, which
influence all the other
systems and organs of
the body.

the HEALTH BENEFITS

Yoga is really good for you. Not only does it stretch the muscles, giving you more flexibility, but it builds your strength and confidence.

It streamlines and tones the body, making you feel well and in control. There are so many benefits – including looking younger.

What's not to like?

Once you've started yoga you'll begin to see the effects on the physical body first – likely within just six weeks.

After balancing the different bodily functions and helping you combat any stiffness or weakness, yoga then moves on to the mental and emotional levels, where it can help you cope with any anxieties too.

YOGA and
CONFIDENCE

Yoga gives you confidence, because when you learn to control and hold the body through your practice, you start to feel more in control of your life. Knowing your body's capabilities gives you confidence in yourself. This is very empowering and it can help you overcome your fears. For example, doing a headstand can be a terrifying prospect at first, but once you recognize the fear and stop wrestling with it, you can take the first steps to doing it. Once you've mastered it, you feel fantastic!

YOGA
and STRESS

Yoga is a way of maintaining health in a stressful society. Practising the various asanas removes physical discomfort, such as after a day hunched over a computer, and the relaxation techniques help minimize stress and give you coping methods when you might normally get upset.

"*Yoga has a sly, clever way of short-circuiting the mental patterns that cause anxiety.*"

BAXTER BELL

"I have been a seeker and I still am, but I stopped asking the books and the stars. I started listening to the teaching of my Soul."

RUMI

YOGA and
emotional TRAUMA

Emotion and stress are stored in the body, which means you may get stiff shoulders, sore hips or a painful back when faced with life's challenges. Yoga can help you to process these feelings and get past them.

A lot of emotions are held in the muscle that goes from the lower spine through the groin to the leg, because it's like an emotional shock-absorber. However, doing hip-opening poses allows the body to release the emotions. Sometimes people are surprised to find that these poses make them cry.

"My biggest struggles have been my biggest teachers."

KATHRYN BUDIG

Another way to release stuck emotion is to open the heart or the chest. By doing back-bending poses you are opening the heart area, and this allows you to release any blocked energy. It's particularly difficult to do this when you feel defensive, but keep your heart open and you will find it easier to forgive and move on.

YOGA and COMMUNITY

An often unforeseen benefit of doing yoga is that it gives you a whole new group of friends. It can take time, but if you go with an open heart you will find good people who are willing to welcome you in. You'll share your experiences and this will bring you together. It's also nice to laugh together at what you can and can't do.

"When the breath wanders, the mind also is unsteady. But when the breath is calmed the mind too will be still, and the yogi achieves long life. Therefore one should learn to control the breath."

HATHA YOGA PRADIPIKA

*"The beauty
is that people often
come here for the
stretch, and leave with
a lot more."*

LIZA CIANO

BODY AWARENESS

With the heightened body awareness that yoga brings, you learn that you can make your own decisions about your body and take responsibility for your health. Yoga often inspires a desire to make healthier choices when eating and a wish to streamline and appreciate the simpler things in life, leading to satisfaction and happiness.

YOGA as THERAPY

Yoga can be used as therapy to regain health after an illness or operation. There are such things as yoga therapists, who will help you to build up strength and stamina after such events. When the body feels depleted, it's also good to get advice from a qualified nutritionist who will tell you what your body needs – but always remember that healing takes time.

"*Sometimes in yoga I feel like a graceful swan. Other times I feel like a baby giraffe trying to use its legs.*"

ANONYMOUS

"No one cares how awesome you look in your postures."

ANONYMOUS

YOGA
on the MOVE

Travelling on a long-haul flight can be eased by doing a few yoga poses while in the queue for the loo. You can exercise pretty much all of the body quite discreetly. Standing on your toes and dropping back onto your feet exercises the calves and keeps the blood flowing. Stretching the arms up and over the head expands the chest and allows more breath to fill the lungs while also stretching out the abdomen. Twists can keep the digestive system from becoming sluggish or getting trapped wind.

YOGA for POSITIVITY

Science says practising yoga allows a better flow of serotonin in the body. Some call this the feel-good brain chemical. With a good flow of serotonin, you can improve your mood and feel more positive.

"Yoga adds years to your life, and life to your years."

ANONYMOUS

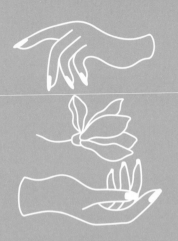

CHAPTER
6

the

BREATH, CHAKRAS and the ENERGETIC BODY

the
BREATH

WHAT IS PRANAYAMA?

Pranayama is defined as breath control. It shows us how to utilize breathing to influence the flow of prana, or life force, in the channels of the energetic body.

This slows the mind down and is extremely beneficial in helping to calm anxieties and lower the blood pressure.

the BENEFITS of PRANAYAMA

The breath is the most vital process of the body. It influences the activities of each cell and is intimately linked with the performance of the brain.

Most people breathe incorrectly, using only a small part of their lung capacity. The breathing is then generally shallow, depriving the body of oxygen and prana, or life force, which is essential for good health.

Rhythmic, deep, slow respiration stimulates calm and creates a content state of mind. Irregular breathing disrupts the rhythms of the brain and leads to physical, emotional and mental blocks.

These in turn lead to inner conflict, an imbalanced personality, a disordered lifestyle and disease.

Pranayama establishes regular breathing patterns, breaking any negative cycles and reversing the process.

It does so by taking control of the breath and re-establishing the natural rhythms of the body and mind. Therefore the energy trapped in neurotic, unconscious mental patterns may be released for use in more creative and joyful activity.

Slow breathing
makes the heart
stronger and
better nourished
and contributes to
a longer life.

PRANAYAMA
for SPIRITUAL
ADVANCEMENT

People seeking spiritual advancement practise pranayama in order to remove blockages in the energetic body (which we will come to in a moment). This increases prana. Many techniques use holding the breath to regulate the flow of prana, calming the mind and controlling the thought process. Once the mind is quiet and prana flows freely, the person will experience higher dimensions of spiritual awareness.

"Yoga begins with listening. When we listen, we are giving space to what is."

RICHARD FREEMAN

the
ENERGETIC
BODY

For centuries, yogis and
healers in several traditions
had a keen understanding
of the physical body,
but also of the
energetic body. They
spoke of energy channels
along which the vital energy
flowed. Many people in
the spiritual field know this
as the aura.

The energetic body refers to the energy field around a person or thing, and just like a set of fingerprints, it's totally unique. These particles of energy are suspended around the healthy human body in an oval-shaped field.

It reaches out about one metre (just over three feet) on all sides and extends above the head and below the feet into the ground. Life was considered a vibrational energy phenomenon, and so health revolved around balancing energy through various means.

"Put your energy into building what is creative, valuable and empowering. And you won't have to constantly fight against what is destructive and draining."

RALPH MARSTON

the AURA

As human beings, we radiate a very low level of electricity that is otherwise known as the electromagnetic field or the aura. It resonates at a certain frequency, and this is what we unconsciously detect in people. Their "energy" may show that they are angry or elated, distraught or excited, and this can be picked up without them having to say a word. Likewise, you will broadcast what you feel to others via your aura.

*"The sensation
of energy expands
with increasing
relaxation."*

ILCHI LEE

ENERGY BLOCKAGES

Energy blockages can occur anywhere, such as in the auras, chakras and the meridian system – channels inside your body that transport energy from one part to another. Meridians have a deep impact on how you think and feel, and your overall health and wellbeing.

These blockages can be caused by many things, including negative thoughts or emotions that have been repressed and that are lodged in the invisible but important bodily energies.

Blockages reduce the flow of energy, creating many different symptoms, including fatigue, low vitality, confusion, slow thinking, a lack of clarity of thought, depression, poor memory and a variety of other symptoms.

Yoga addresses these energy blocks by moving the body, stretching and working the meridians, which rebalances the flow of energy.

"In every culture and in every medical tradition before ours, healing was accomplished by moving energy."

ALBERT SZENT-GYÖRGYI
Biochemist and Nobel Prize-Winner

the
CHAKRAS

The chakras are invisible, whirling vortices of energy located at certain points in the body.

They control the circulation of prana and are connected to the aura. Each chakra is a doorway that opens up specific areas of the brain.

In most people these psychic centres lie dormant and inactive, so concentrating on the chakras while performing yogic practices stimulates the flow of energy and helps to activate them.

This allows you to experience the higher planes of consciousness that are normally inaccessible.

There are seven chakras, each with a Sanskrit name and a different colour associated with it, and specific yoga poses can be used to harmonize and balance each one.

BASE or ROOT CHAKRA - MULADHARA

colour: deep red

The first and lowest of the chakras is situated at the base of the body, and is known as the root chakra. It is related to survival, our place on the earth and our security. If blocked, you may experience paranoia, insecurity, or a feeling of being out of touch with reality.

SACRAL CHAKRA - SVADHISTHANA

colour: orange

Situated two fingers above the root chakra in the spine behind the genital organs, this chakra is related to sensuality, sexuality and the desire for pleasure. If blocked, you may experience emotional issues, sexual problems or unsettling emotions. If it's too open, you may be into sexually addictive, manipulative or excessive behaviour.

SOLAR PLEXUS CHAKRA
- MANIPURA

colour: yellow

Situated just behind the navel in the spine, this chakra is related to our ability to wield power in this world. It can be called "the fire in the belly" and it is the centre of self-assertion, dynamism and dominance. When in balance, it allows you to control your destiny, feel your power and accomplish your dreams. Negatively, it can result in obsessive-compulsive control.

HEART CHAKRA
- ANAHATA
colour: green

Situated in the spine behind the sternum and level with the heart, this chakra relates to love and compassion, because it operates from the heart centre. This is where feelings of universal brotherhood and tolerance begin to develop and all beings are accepted and loved for what they are. Healthy relationships, pets, family, beauty and nature enhance the health of this chakra.

THROAT
CHAKRA
- VISHUDDHA

colour: blue

The throat chakra is where you say what you believe to be true. When this chakra is flowing at optimum levels, you are able to ask for what you need. If you find it hard to speak up or say what you really mean, then singing, chanting and breathing exercises can enhance the health of this chakra.

THIRD EYE CHAKRA

- AJNA

colour: indigo

This chakra is situated on the forehead between the eyebrows. It corresponds with the pineal gland. This is where wisdom and intuition develop. When activated, the mind becomes steady, strong and in full control. When blocked, there will be a lack of insight, awareness or guidance.

CROWN CHAKRA
- SAHASRARA

colour: white or violet

The crown chakra is located at the top of the head, and it represents our ability to be fully connected spiritually. A fully open crown chakra enables you to access your higher consciousness.

"The more willing you are to surrender to the energy within you, the more power can flow through you."

SHAKTI GAWAIN

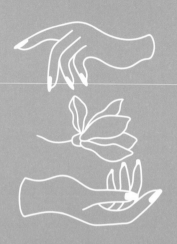

CHAPTER
7

using
SOUND
in YOGA

You may come across sound
being used in yoga, usually
as part of the meditation
process. Although this chapter
touches on sound healing, it
is worth mentioning that yoga
and sound work really well
together. There may be calming
music playing during a class,
or you may be encouraged
to chant. Don't let the fear of
making a sound put you off.

Sound affects every cell in our bodies and works on all levels: emotional, physical and spiritual. Many people have reported that they feel more relaxed, less stressed and sleep better after a few sound-healing sessions.

It is also believed that sound healing removes blockages and toxins.

Sound healing does not require any medication and there are no side effects. When combined with yoga, it can be especially effective.

MEDITATION

Meditation is about slowing the mind to a place of "no thought". Once you can meditate, you can master your thoughts and then master your life. It prevents your emotions from running wild and you will find you are calmer and happier as a result. You can meditate silently or with sound. Meditating after a yoga session is likely to be successful because the body is relaxed and the mind is quiet at that time.

MANTRAS

Mantras are sometimes used in yoga classes to help with meditation. A mantra is a series of phrases or words that are sung or chanted during meditation. They are formulae that alter the patterns of the mind and the chemistry of the brain.
A mantra is more than a repeated phrase, because it is the energy created by the chanting or singing that makes the phrase a mantra.

Repeated sufficiently, a mantra can shift a thought or concept into the subconscious level of the mind. Mantras are energy vibrations of repeated sounds. They can be sung, whispered or said in thought only. One example is:

Om mane padme hum.

HOW DO MANTRAS HELP?

Repeating a mantra stops the mind from wandering. It produces a rhythm and a flow that is easy for the mind to grasp. When the mind gets distracted, the mantra helps bring it back. The rhythm of the mantra provides an easy channel for energy to flow in and out. For some, knowing the meaning of the mantra can improve its effectiveness.

do you
NEED to KNOW
what the
MANTRA MEANS?

The meaning of the mantra itself has no power; it is the vibration it creates in the body that matters. These vibrations have neuro-linguistic effects that evoke a feeling of calm, and they are said to help people with serious diseases who suffer from hopelessness to feel more optimistic again.

the PHYSICAL BENEFITS of MANTRAS

The rhythm and sound of the chanting moves energy throughout the body and this regulates the chemicals in our brain, lowering the effect of stress hormones while simultaneously releasing the "feel-good" endorphins. Mantras lower the heart rate and blood pressure, while enhancing positive brainwaves and increasing immune functions.

The sound of the mantra
literally drowns out the
negative voices in our heads.
When negative thoughts are
suppressed, the mind has
room for positive thoughts, so
it is an easy way to improve
mental health. Mantras ease
fear, so people with phobias
often use them as something
to focus on when they
are afraid.

TIBETAN SINGING BOWLS

You may not be familiar with Tibetan singing bowls, but you might have seen or heard them in a meditation or yoga class. Tibetan singing bowls have been used for centuries for healing and meditation purposes, because they create a range of sounds that restore the normal vibratory frequencies of diseased and out-of-harmony parts of the body, mind and soul.

The pure sonic waves that ring from Tibetan singing bowls enhance our ability to hear with more than our ears. We *feel* the sound of Tibetan singing bowls as much as we hear it.

"If we accept that sound is vibration and we know that vibration touches every part of our physical being, then we understand that sound is heard not only through our ears but through every cell in our bodies. One reason sound heals on a physical level is because it so deeply touches and transforms us on the emotional and spiritual planes. Sound can redress imbalances on every level of physiological functioning, and can play a positive role in the treatment of virtually any medical disorder."

DR MITCHELL GAYNOR

director of Medical Oncology & Integrative Medicine, the
Cornell Cancer Prevention Center in New York

GONG HEALING

Gong healing is an ancient practice which can access deep states of meditation and balance. It brings the mind to a state of clarity and neutrality, which can enhance creativity. The vibration of the gong puts pressure on the nervous system to adjust and heal itself, thus acting as a reset button for the entire body. The sound opens up the energy pathways and penetrates every cell in the body, removing blocks and tension, bringing the body and mind into a state of deep relaxation for healing and rejuvenation.

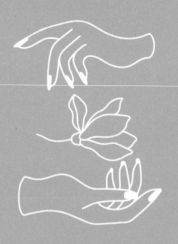

CHAPTER

8

your FIRST YOGA CLASS

WHAT
TO KNOW

before you go

- Anyone can be a yogi

- You don't need to move to India or join a yoga studio to practise yoga

- You can't be bad at yoga. Nobody is bad at yoga

- Practise patience. Yoga is a lifelong rehearsal

- There is not a one-size-fits-all yoga practice

- Always look at your practice with a beginner's mind

ARRIVE EARLY

Get to the class at least ten minutes before the scheduled time, in case there's paperwork to fill out or you want to ask about anything. Arriving early also gives you a chance to find a spot for your mat and connect with the teacher. Be sure to say it's your first time.

THERE MIGHT BE CHANTING

Some classes like to chant at the beginning or the end of a class. If you're not comfortable with this, there's no pressure to take part. Just breathe, relax and keep an open mind. If you do join in, don't worry about getting the chant exactly right.

RELEASE the TENSION

You may not realize that you're tense when you first start your class, but the more you let go and release this stress from your body, the easier every pose will feel. Focusing on the breathing will help you stay relaxed and allow you to have a better experience. Once you've chilled out, you'll find that you're able to hold poses for longer.

DON'T WORRY

about being a

BEGINNER

In only six weeks or so you will have a much clearer idea of what you're doing. In yoga practice, the idea of a beginner's mind means you have no preconceived notions about what you can or can't do. Keeping this positive outlook and leaving expectations at the door will result in the best experience possible.

CHILD'S POSE
is always an option

If ever you feel the need to stop, if you are tired or overwhelmed, you can always take up Child's Pose (shown opposite).

This pose will help you to "zen out" and tune into your body's needs.

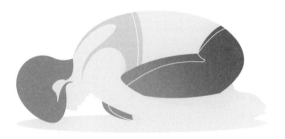

Child's Pose

TRUST the TEACHER

Your teacher's pace might be difficult for you at the outset. However, trust their choice of poses and do your best to follow the sequence. You can always stop and rejoin when you're ready. Also know that some teachers are more hands-on than others. If you're not comfortable with what is going on, please tell your instructor.

COMMUNICATE
with your
TEACHER

Tell them of any injuries or conditions you have and what's going on for you, because that helps them to help you.

WEAR LOOSE, COMFORTABLE CLOTHES

and remove glasses, watches
and jewellery

RELAX!

YOGA

should be

ENJOYABLE

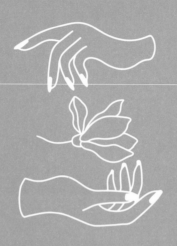

CHAPTER

9

some
FINAL
ADVICE

DON'T
COMPARE
YOURSELF
to OTHERS

It's not helpful and only leads to negative thinking. We are all different and on our own journeys.

BREATH is EVERYTHING

Usually the teacher will tell you when to inhale or exhale with a movement. This helps you to forget about life outside the class for a while and to relax. Pay attention to how shallow your breath is at the beginning of the class and notice if it's deeper and more relaxed by the end.

have a
SENSE
of HUMOUR

Although yoga is a quiet, focused activity,
don't take it too seriously. Humility and
the ability to laugh allow things to flow in
our lives much more easily, and you will
find it more enjoyable and liberating.

find a
TEACHER
who is
RIGHT
for YOU

if you don't like the teacher, find another
one, because you must feel comfortable
with the class vibe.

DON'T do YOGA on a FULL STOMACH

Doing yoga straight after mealtimes will hinder your practice, and you can't work while your stomach is busy digesting something heavy. It's best to eat at least an hour beforehand and make this a light snack, but if you are hungry, eat a banana no less than twenty minutes before a class.

LEAVE YOUR EGO at the DOOR

This isn't a competitive sport and no one else really cares whether you can touch your toes or not! This is your journey and nothing to do with anyone else

ALWAYS
LISTEN
to your BODY

If any poses hurt, then come out of them immediately and do so carefully.

MODIFY
POSTURES
for your **BODY...**

and don't worry about trying to do the
perfect pose.

JUST
BREATHE

Yoga is not just about physical exercise.
It helps to establish a new way of life
which embraces inner and outer realities.

This is something you cannot learn
intellectually – it becomes living knowledge
through practice and experience.

TIME

Yoga can be done at any time, but according to ancient texts, the best time is two hours before and including sunrise. This is because the atmosphere is pure and quiet and the activities of the stomach and intestines haven't started for the day and the mind is empty of thoughts.

In the evening, an hour either side of sunset is optimal.

START by working with WHAT YOU HAVE

Respect your body's inner wisdom and limitations and don't do anything that feels wrong for you.

PRACTICE
in a **WELL-VENTILATED ROOM**
that is calm and quiet

YOGA can become
ADDICTIVE

Once you realize how good you feel afterwards, you will naturally want more of it. Remember, however, that you must keep things in balance in order to protect yourself from injury.

Unfortunately, an unbridled ego can push you too far and that is when you can hurt yourself, so you need to be mindful of what you're doing.

DRINK lots of WATER

Make sure you have plenty of water available to drink after a yoga session, as this helps to flush out toxins in the body that have been moved around during the session.

CONCLUSION

remember: it's never too late to start yoga.

It doesn't matter how old you are or how unfit; it's a journey that gets better the further you go.

"Namaste."